10/04

S0-AJM-498

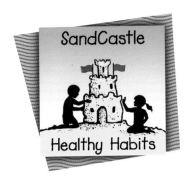

SandCastle

Healthy Habits

Being Active

Mary Elizabeth Salzmann

Consulting Editor, Diane Craig, M.A./Reading Specialist

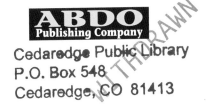

ABDO
Publishing Company

Published by ABDO Publishing Company, 4940 Viking Drive, Edina, Minnesota 55435.

Credits
Edited by: Pam Price
Curriculum Coordinator: Nancy Tuminelly
Cover and Interior Design and Production: Mighty Media
Photo Credits: BananaStock Ltd., Digital Vision, Image 100, Image Source, ImageState, Stockbyte

Library of Congress Cataloging-in-Publication Data

Salzmann, Mary Elizabeth, 1968-
      Being active / Mary Elizabeth Salzmann.
          p. cm. -- (Healthy habits)
      Includes index.
      Summary: Explains in simple language the importance of regular physical activity.
      ISBN 1-59197-550-6
      1. Exercise for children--Juvenile literature. 2. Physical fitness for children--Juvenile literature. 3. Children--Health and hygiene--Juvenile literature. [1. Exercise. 2. Physical fitness.] I. Title.

RJ133.S24 2004
613.7'042--dc22
                                                                    2003057789

SandCastle™ books are created by a professional team of educators, reading specialists, and content developers around five essential components that include phonemic awareness, phonics, vocabulary, text comprehension, and fluency. All books are written, reviewed, and leveled for guided reading, early intervention reading, and Accelerated Reader® programs and designed for use in shared, guided, and independent reading and writing activities to support a balanced approach to literacy instruction.

Let Us Know

After reading the book, SandCastle would like you to tell us your stories about reading. What is your favorite page? Was there something hard that you needed help with? Share the ups and downs of learning to read. We want to hear from you! To get posted on the ABDO Publishing Company Web site, send us e-mail at:

sandcastle@abdopub.com

SandCastle Level: Transitional

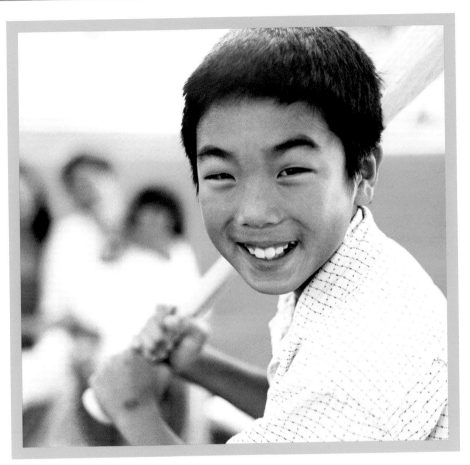

Being active is
a healthy habit.

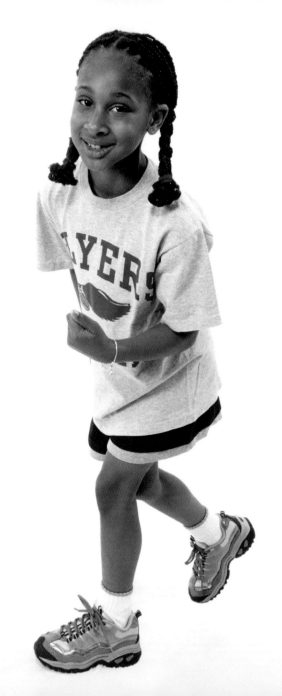

Being active helps your muscles grow strong.

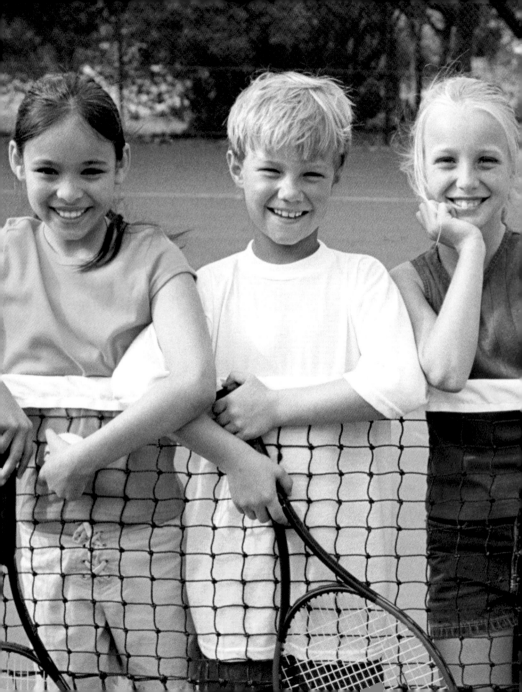

Being active also helps you feel happy and good about yourself.

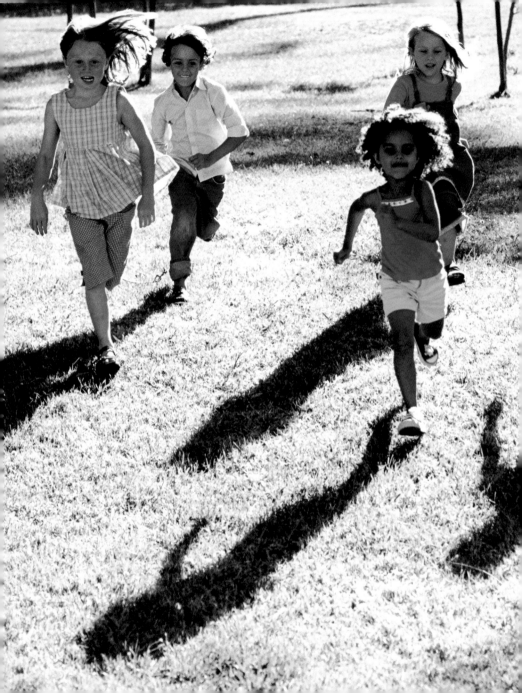

It is important to be active for at least a little while every day.

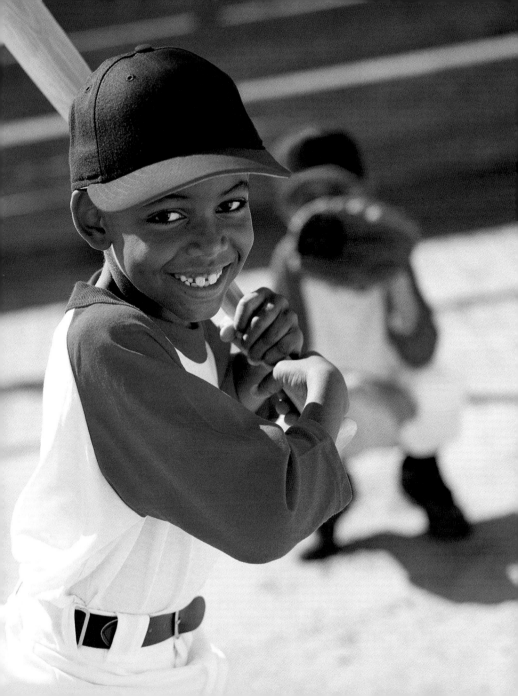

Ken plays on a
baseball team.

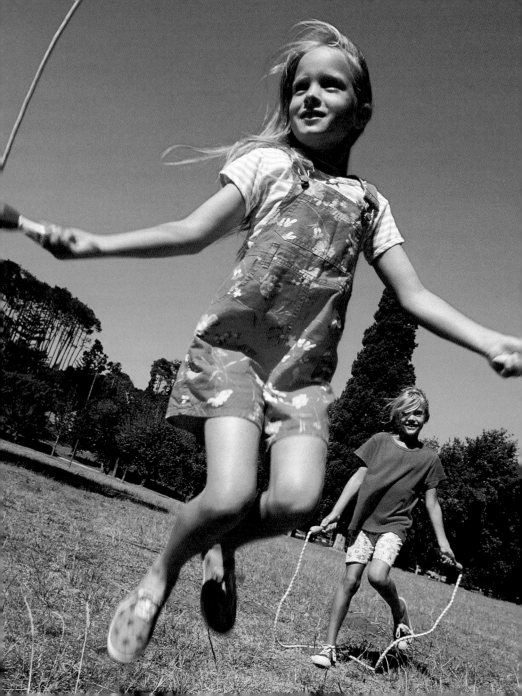

Molly and Nina like to jump rope.

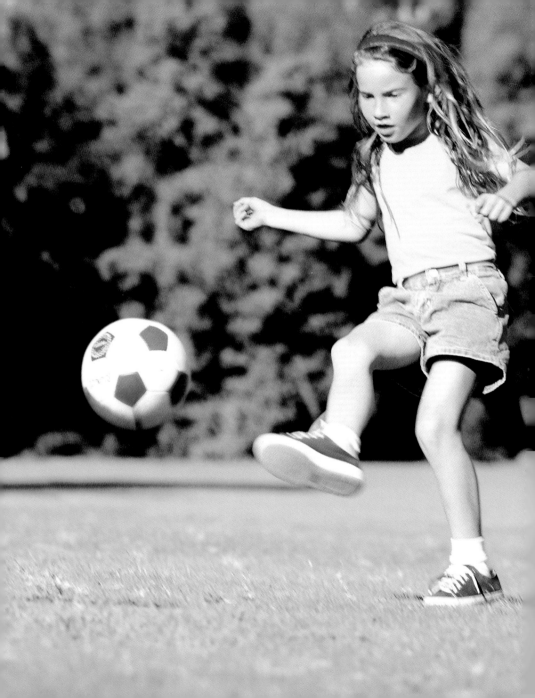

Sue plays soccer after school.

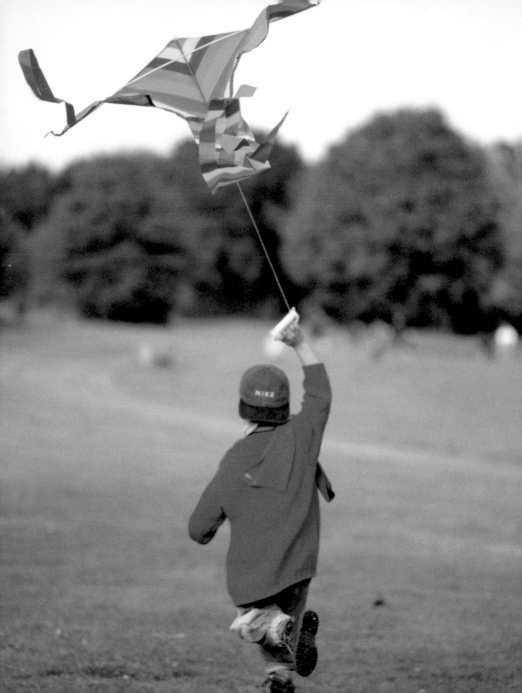

Jake flies his kite in the park.

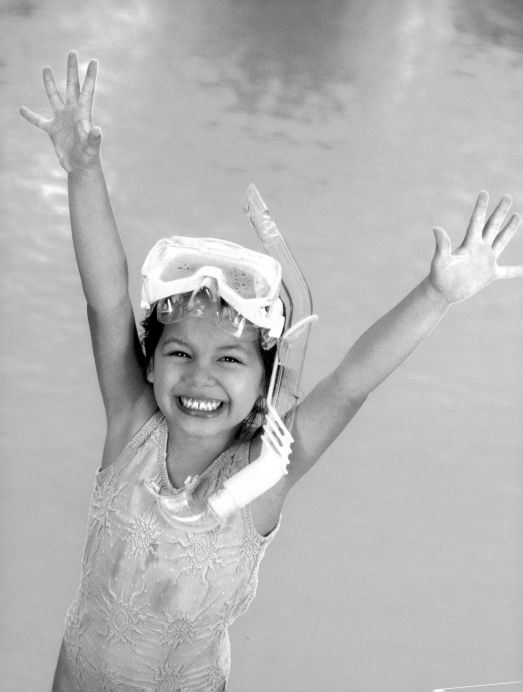

Lisa loves to swim in the summertime.

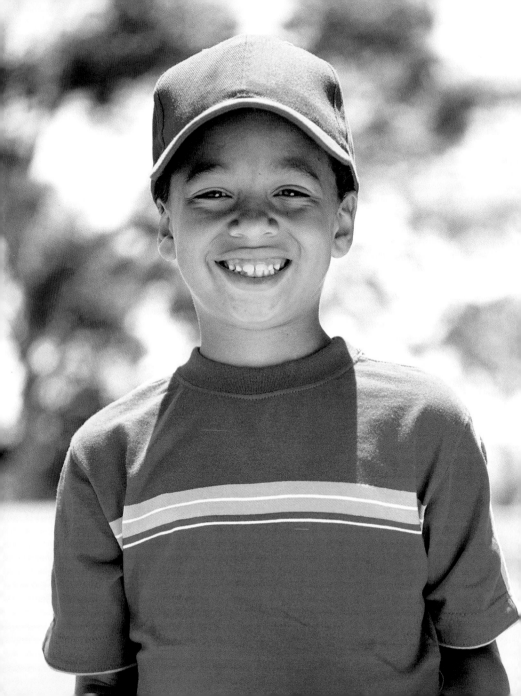

What is your favorite way to be active?

Did You Know?

You have 650 muscles in your body.

Little League baseball is the world's largest youth sports organization.

In 1989 Park Bong-tae of South Korea jumped rope 14,628 times in one hour.

Soccer is called football in most countries outside the United States.

The largest kite ever flown was 210 feet long and 72 feet wide. It flew for almost 23 minutes in 1997.

Glossary

baseball. a game played with a bat and ball on a field with four bases marking the path the players must run in order to score

habit. a behavior done so often that it becomes automatic

healthy. preserving the wellness of body, mind, or spirit

kite. a lightweight frame covered with paper or fabric that is flown at the end of a long string

muscle. the body tissue connected to the bones that allows us to move

soccer. a game played by two teams that try to get the ball into the other team's goal without touching it with their hands or arms

About SandCastle™

A professional team of educators, reading specialists, and content developers created the SandCastle™ series to support young readers as they develop reading skills and strategies and increase their general knowledge. The SandCastle™ series has four levels that correspond to early literacy development in young children. The levels are provided to help teachers and parents select the appropriate books for young readers.

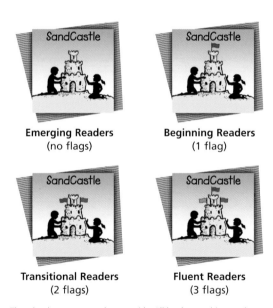

Emerging Readers
(no flags)

Beginning Readers
(1 flag)

Transitional Readers
(2 flags)

Fluent Readers
(3 flags)

These levels are meant only as a guide. All levels are subject to change.

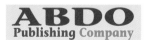

To see a complete list of SandCastle™ books and other nonfiction titles from ABDO Publishing Company, visit **www.abdopub.com** or contact us at:

4940 Viking Drive, Edina, Minnesota 55435 • 1-800-800-1312 • fax: 1-952-831-1632